Summer Diffusers:

Super Refreshing Recipes for Cooling and Calming on a Hot Summer

Table of Content:

Introduction

In the fast-paced world of today, many of us find that there is something missing in our life. As we go through the motions, we feel an almost imperceptible but nagging impulse that we are lacking something.

Many find themselves racked with anxiety, depression, or simply a lack of energy. Well, if that's the case, I've got some good news for you because the age-old practice of diffusing oils just might be what the doctor ordered.

Call it aromatherapy or just plain oil diffusion, it all amounts to the same thing—results! Most just don't realize how powerful of an instrument our nose is. But whether we realize it or not, the nose is an important gateway to our brain. It is the nose that sorts through all the chemical data that comes our day every single day.

Whether this chemical data is from the smell of a juicy cheeseburger you are about to eat or the stench of the doggy poop you just stepped in outside.

All of these things, whether pleasant, or not so pleasant, are providing our brain important sensory information. It is our nose inhaling this aroma that interfaces with our brain in order to provoke an appropriate physiological reaction. But along with simply reading information, our brain can actually be therapeutically charged by the stimulus that we literally breathe into it.

Your nose is much more important than you ever realized you see, and as the gateway to physiological change, the idea that you can harness this powerful tool in order to directly alter or enhance mood, energy, and even the immune system—is a real game changer.

As you read this book you will find many ways that you can make the best of this biological fine tuner. You will find essential oil-based recipes that you can put into a simple diffuser in order to facilitate any desired change in temperament. And that my friends, is news you can use, and most certainly—news you can diffuse!

Chapter 1: Diffusers for the Mind

The mind is a terrible thing to waste, yet many of us fret and fritter away our minds on worry, stress, and depression on a daily basis. Here in this chapter we provide for you recipes that will clear the skies of your mental fog.

You no longer have to be stuck in the incessant doldrums of lackluster and lethargy. Employ the recipes presented in this chapter and soon you will be feeling just fine. You've just got to check out some of these sure-fire, guaranteed, diffusers for the mind.

Anxiety Busting Diffuser Recipe

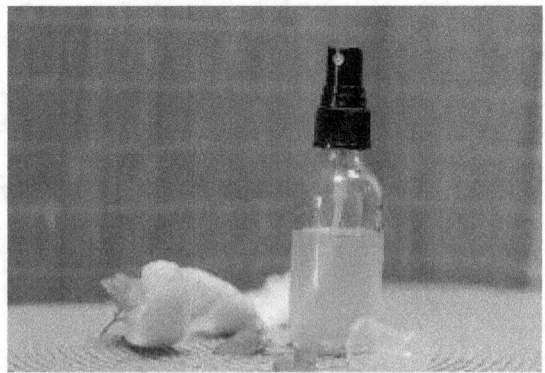

Anxiety in the modern world has increased to something akin to epidemic like proportions. People are anxious for politics, finances, relationships—you name it, and there is some way to be anxious about it!

In the high-pressure cooking world of today we sometimes feel like we're getting thoroughly baked as we pass through, but just a couple drops of lavender mixed with clary sage, and bergamot.

You see, because although what tomorrow may hold is anyone's guess—with this great anxiety busting diffuser, you can have quite a leg up on the rest! Try out this diffuser recipe so that you can always be at your absolute best!

Here are the exact ingredients:

2 drops of lavender essential oil

3 drops of clary sage essential oil

3 drops of bergamot essential oil

1 cup of water

The scent of bergamot is pleasing to the senses. Upon smelling this citrus scent most just think that it "smells good". But the soothing feeling of bergamot runs deeper than even its feel-good fresh fragrance, because the aroma of bergamot carries within it a special compound called Linalyl Acetate.

This is an element found in many essential oil blends since it is so good at reducing inflammation and promoting a general sense of relaxation. Couple this with a couple drops of soothing lavender and a few drops of clary sage and you have got it made in the shade!

Just mix all the above-mentioned ingredients together with 1 cup of water in your oil base, and deposit into a diffuser. Allow the aroma to fill the room and you will soon see some fairly tremendous results when it comes to reducing the onset and severity of any anxiety you may face. So, get ready to try this powerful recipe out for yourself!

Depression Easing Diffuser

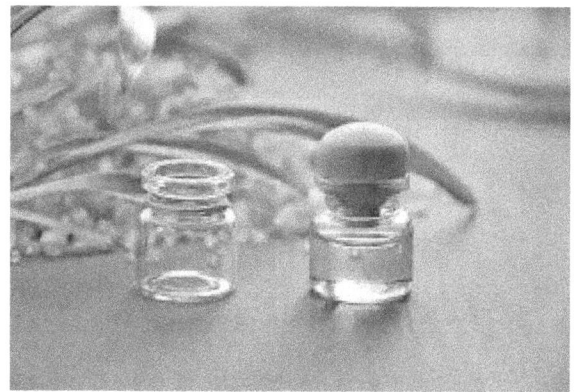

Feeling a bit depressed? Don't worry. It's completely natural to have the blues from time to time. Depression can sneak up on us when we least expect it. It is exceedingly good therefore, to have a depression easing diffuser like this one on hand to combat those gloomy dispositions.

Just take a few whiffs of this diffuser and you will sing the blues no more! This blend of jasmine, rose, and frankincense essential oil is a tremendous variety of health in healing at your disposal.

Here are the exact ingredients:

3 drops of jasmine essential oil

2 drops of rose essential oil

3 drops of frankincense essential oil

1 cup of water

In order to create a strong blend of the above-mentioned ingredients, you are going to need to add your cup of water, followed by your 3 drops of jasmine, 2 drops of rose, and 3 drops of frankincense to a plastic container.

After mixing together, place a lid on the container and manually shake everything up even further. Now add your mixture to a diffuser, set it out in the middle of a room, and breathe in the aroma.

After just a couple of hours you should begin to feel the difference. So, if you need a lift in your mood, this diffuser just might be for you.

Fixing Your Focus Diffuser

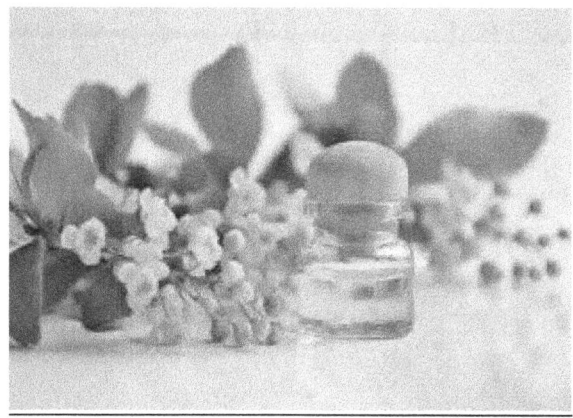

Sometimes we can get so distracted that even on one of our best days being able to hold onto our concentration can be incredibly difficult. We have a lot of challenges that we may face throughout our day, but regaining your focus and clarity does not have to be a mission impossible.

And this essential oil cocktail proves it. With this blend of oils, you will be able to hold your focus for longer periods of time even while you improve your memory and ability to recall information.

Here are the exact ingredients:

4 drops of cypress essential oil

3 drops of rosemary essential oil

4 drops of coriander essential oil

1 cup of water

Add your cup of water followed by your 4 drops of cypress oil, 3 drops of rosemary oil, and 4 drops of coriander oil to a container, and stir it all together well.

After this initial stirring, place a lid on top and the shake contents well. After this, pour the mixture into your diffuser and allow it to take hold, letting the scent slowly waft through your home. Try to breathe in as deeply as possible and your focus will be improved in no time at all.

Confidence Building Diffuser

In this uncertain world, many of us can have issues with our confidence from time to time. This confidence building diffuser does just that.

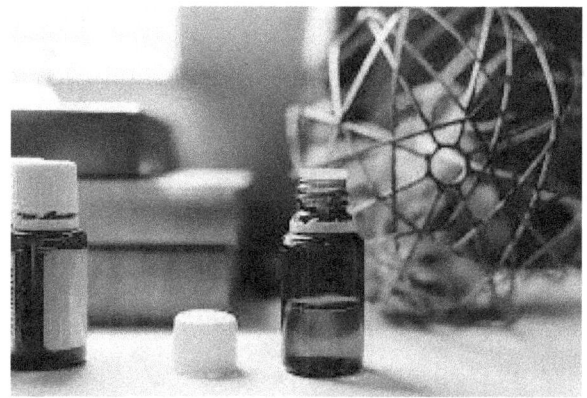

Just breathe in the soothing and powerful scent of frankincense, rosemary, and sweet orange, and you will your courage begin to grow! It doesn't matter where you are or what you are doing. This herbal mood booster will keep you well, and get you right out onto the ground floor!

Here are the exact ingredients:

4 drops of frankincense essential oil

3 drops of rosemary essential oil

4 drops of sweet orange essential oil

1 cup of water

Get out a medium sized mixing bowl and add your cup of water followed by your 4 drops of sweet orange, 3 drops of rosemary, and your 4 drops frankincense.

You will see the water color and quality begin to change. Stir all of the ingredients together and pour into a diffuser. Allow aroma to fil the room and gradually breathe in the confidence building aroma.

Chapter 2: Diffusers for Summer Allergies

Summer is a time to kick back, relax, and enjoy the sunshine. But its also a time when seasonal allergies are at their height. Just about every plant known to man is in bloom this time of year, and that means heavy pollen counts and an increased incidence of sneezing and watery eyes can most certainly be expected.

But don't let these summertime allergy blues get the best of you—just get a dose of some of these great diffusers for summer allergies.

Hay Fever Blocking Diffuser

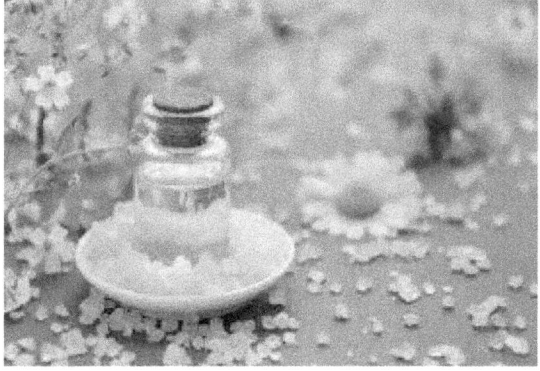

Hay fever triggered by pollen can be a real downer during the summer months. It can be a real hassle when every single time you go outside your nose swells up like a balloon and then simultaneously drips like a faucet

But this hay fever blocking diffuser holds the promise of keeping even the worst of your hay fever symptoms at bay. So don't suffer a second longer—try this recipe today!

Here are the exact ingredients:

3 drops of peppermint essential oil

2 drops of eucalyptus essential oil

3 drops of lavender essential oil

1 cup of water

To start off this refreshing diffuser blend, add a up of water to a medium sized mixing bowl. After you have done this you can then add in your 3 drops of peppermint oil, your 2 drops of eucalyptus oil, and your 3 drops of lavender oil. Mix everything together well and allow to sit for a few minutes.

You will see the liquid congeal into a nice and thick consistency once it all settles in place. After this, pour it all into your diffuser and let the aroma gently fill the room. And you will feel better soon.

Poison Oak/Ivy Soothing Diffuser

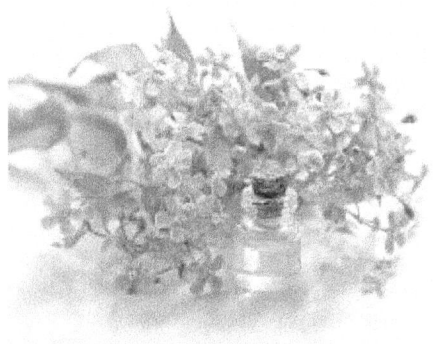

That itchy, burning feeling of being subjected to poison oak or ivy is hard to deal with. But what if you could ease some of the suffering with a few rounds of aromatherapy? The good news is that you can! You see, much of the effects of poison oak and ivy are caused by our own body's reaction to the oils from these plants.

If we can get our body's reaction under control therefore, then we have won half the battle right there. With its anti-inflammatory properties to bring down swelling, itchiness and hives, this poison oak/ivy soothing diffuser does just that.

If you find yourself haphazardly walking into the midst of poison oak and ivy, don't panic, just reach for this poison oak/ivy soothing diffuser.

Because a batch of this essential oil blend can do you a world of good when it comes to influencing how your body reacts to the harmful chemicals released by these plants. So, don't go camping without it!

Here are the exact ingredients:

½ cup of hot water

1 tsp of sea salt

¼ cup of apple cider vinegar

3 drops of lavender essential oil

2 drops of eucalyptus essential oil

Get out a medium sized mixing bowl and deposit your ½ cup of hot water into the bottom of it. Follow this by adding your ¼ cup of cider vinegar. Stir your water and vinegar together well before adding in your 1 tsp of sea salt.

After this, add your 3 drops of lavender oil and your 2 drops of eucalyptus oil. Mix all of these ingredients together thoroughly and allow to sit out for a few minutes.

Once everything has settled, go ahead and put the ingredients into your diffuser and set out in the middle of the room so that you can slowly inundate yourself with the aroma.

By breathing in these vapors your body will relax and allow the initial swelling of the breakout to go down. After the swelling goes down the body will generally relax, and begin the healing process of the skin.

Pollen Neutralizing Oil Mix

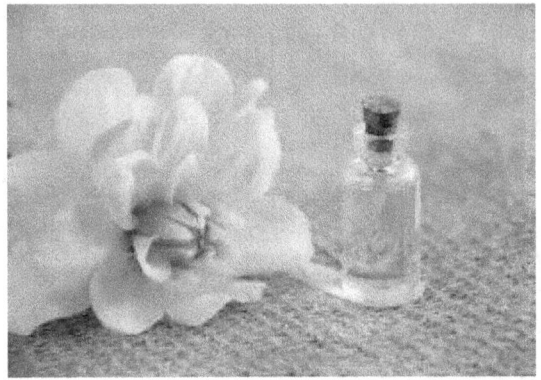

Pollen can be a real bummer if you have to be outside during the summer months. And if you are especially sensitive to pollen allergens it could be downright miserable with itchy, watery eyes, runny nose, skin broken out in hives and the like.

This is certainly no way to spend your summer! Who wants to be embarrassed and broken out during a trip to the swimming pool? The simple answer is—no one. It's just that most don't know how to counteract their allergic reactions to pollen effectively.

Having that said, pay especially close attention to the following recipe since it offers a potential way around this some of these allergen triggers. You need to nip the pollen in the bud, and you can do it with this special pollen neutralizing oil mix!

Here are the exact ingredients:

12 drops of peppermint essential oil

12 drops of lavender essential oil

12 drops of lemon essential oil

1 cup or water

To get this batch going, get out a medium sized mixing bowl or container and add your cup of water. Follow this up by adding your 12 drops of peppermint oil, your 12 drops of lavender oil, and your 12 drops of lemon oil.

Stir everything together well until it constitutes a fine mixture. After you have done this, leave the mix out on the counter to settle for a few minutes.

You are now free to pour the mixture into your diffuser and allow the aroma to slowly accumulate throughout your living area. Slowly but surely you will be inundated with the benefits of this pollen neutralizing oil mix.

All-Natural Anti Histamine Diffuser

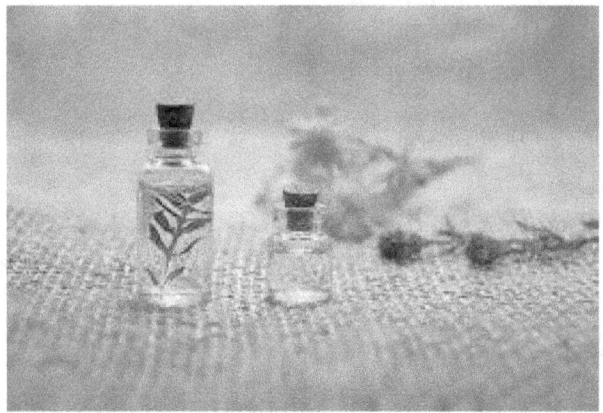

This all-natural anti histamine diffuser really does its work! Loaded with peppermint, lavender and lemon essential oil, it puts over the counter anti histamines to shame! If you are feeling even the least bit under the weather this allergy season you should give this remedy a try!

5 drops of peppermint essential oil

4 drops of lavender essential oil

4 drops of lemon essential oil

1 cup of water

Get out a large mixing bowl or container and add your cup of water to it. After this add your 5 drops of peppermint oil, followed by your 4 drops of lavender oil, and your 4 drops of lemon oil.

This will give you a powerful citrus based but also flowery blend for your diffuser. Stir everything together well before leaving the mixture out at room temperatures for a few minutes so that it can settle in place.

After you have done this, pour the mix into your diffuser, activate it, and allow the healing and therapeutic aroma to fill the room. You'll be feeling better soon!

Chapter 3: Diffusers for Immune Health

The immune system is not something that we can take for granted. Without an immune system we could quite literally die of a cold. As evidenced by the rare few that are born into this world with a compromised immune system and have to be careful of every single germ, they encounter.

If you have ever seen the movie the "Bubble Boy" then you have borne witness to what it might be like to live without a proper immune system to provide your defense.

Essentially, we would indeed have to live in a bubble in order to avoid getting sick. Thankfully for most of us, our biology gives us a natural, invisible bubble that surrounds us and when our immune system is healthy it can block out and repel almost all of the germs that we may encounter.

So, if your immune system is a bit sluggish or lacking you might want to check out this chapter and what it can do for you're the overall state of your immune health.

Immune Boosting Diffuser Combo

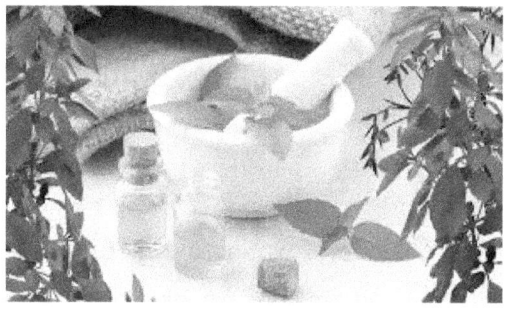

If your immune system is in need of a boost, the soothing oils of this aromatic diffuser combo will help put your immune system right back on track where it needs to be. Sometimes we need that little bit of an extra push to get us going.

This immune boosting diffuser combo does just that. If you feel like your immune system could use just a little bit of help to go the extra mile, give this immune boosting recipe a try!

Here are the exact ingredients:

12 drops of essential eucalyptus oil

12 drops of essential frankincense oil

12 drops of essential rosemary oil

12 drops of essential lemon oil

1 cup of water

First off, add your cup of water to a medium sized mixing bowl. After this, add in your 12 drops of eucalyptus oil, followed by your 12 drops of frankincense oil, your 12 drops of rosemary oil, and your 12 drops of lemon oil. Stir everything together well and add to your diffuser. Turn on, and slowly acclimate yourself with the aroma.

Heart Health Diffuser

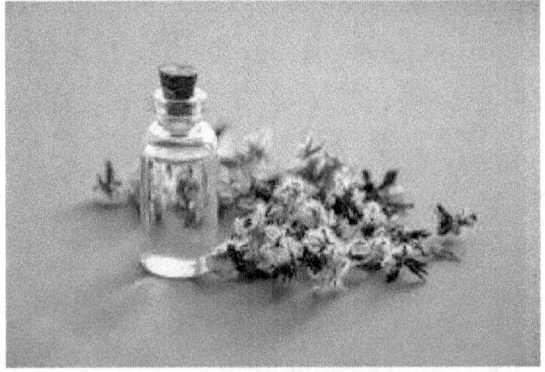

The heart is our most vital organ. Simply put, if the heart goes out on us, the rest of our body doesn't stand much of a chance. Having that said, we could all use a little bit of help when it comes to the health of our heart. In order to make sure that your heart is beating nice and strong. You just might want to check out this tremendous blend of heart health diffuser.

Here are the exact ingredients:

4 drops of peppermint essential oil

5 drops of lemon essential oil

2 drops of basil essential oil

2 cups of water

This recipe brings together peppermint, lemon, and basil to provide a powerful blend of heart boosting elements. Basil provides a dose of magnesium to improve the pumping of blood, while peppermint and lemon get the immune system to jumpstart your arteries. Having that said, in order to give your heart a solid boost, just add 2 cups of water to a large bowl followed by 4 drops of peppermint oil and 5 drops of lemon oil.

Stir these ingredients together well and give them a moment to settle in at room temperature. After this sprinkle your 2 drops of basil oil on top and mix everything together well. Place in a diffuser and you are good to go.

Healthy Metabolism Diffuser

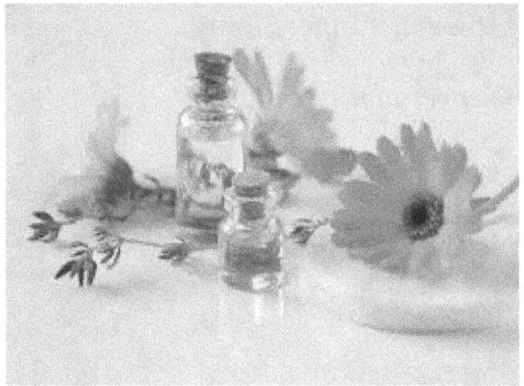

If you ever need to lose weight, you can now how hard it can be—especially if you have trouble with a slow metabolism. But a healthy metabolism is important not just for weight loss, it's an integral part of holistic health altogether. Here in this recipe you will find the means to give your metabolism a boost.

Here are the exact ingredients:

4 drops of clove essential oil

2 drops of citrus essential oil

1 drop of lemon essential oil

1 cup of water

Get out a medium sized mixing bowl or small container and add your cup of water. Next put your 4 drops of clove oil in place. After this settles in, add your 2 drops of citrus oil, and your drop of lemon oil.

Stir everything together well and add to your diffuser. Allow the aroma to permeate your living quarters and breathe in the fragrance over the next few days. Soon enough you will see the results of a lower, slower, and much healthier metabolism.

Germ Guard Diffuser

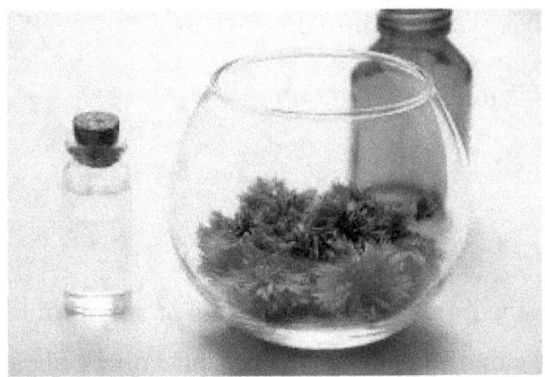

If you are around germs a lot, such as would be the case if you work at a hospital, nursing home, or perhaps even a public school—you may want to gird yourself with this special germ guard diffuser. This blend will help your body keep a proactive edge when it comes to keeping germs at bay.

Here are the exact ingredients:

2 drops of lemon essential oil

3 drops of citrus essential oil

5 drops of orange essential oil

3 drops of clove essential oil

1 cup of water

For this one, place your water into the mixing bowl first, followed by your 2 drops of lemon oil, your 3 drops of citrus oil, and your 5 drops of orange oil. Stir everything together well and allow the ingredients to settle for a few moments at room temp.

Once this has been established add the final ingredient— your 3 drops of clove oil. Stir and mix all of the ingredients together thoroughly before depositing into your diffuser. This citrusy blend will then fill the room and your lungs, empowering you with a special defense against all those germs that may be flitting about.

Regular immersions in these healthy vapors will certainly give you an edge during the cold and flu seasons. This blend disinfects even as it invigorates. Use as often as necessary.

Classic Immune Boosting Diffuser

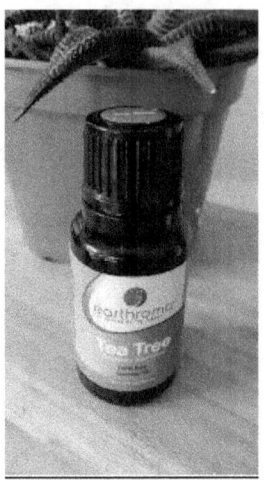

This diffuser has a classic ability when it comes to boosting the immune system. The lemon essential oil gives the body a disinfectant protecting edge while eucalyptus generally increase the body's ability to heal.

Here are the exact ingredients:

5 drops of thrive essential oil

5 drops of eucalyptus essential oil

5 drops of tea tree essential oil

5 drops of lemon essential oil

2 cups of water

First, fill your diffuser with your two cups of water. Next, add your 5 drops of lemon oil followed by your 5 drops of eucalyptus oil, and 5 drops of thrive oil.

After this, you can plug in your diffuser and adjust the temp and humidity of the device to the appropriate setting. Finally add your 5 drops of tea tree oil.

You are now ready to breathe in the healing aroma of this classic immune boosting diffuser. Just steadily breathe in the fragrance over the next few hours. Here's to your immune health!

Chapter 4: Diffusers for Energy and Emotional Wellbeing

We could all use a little bit of a boost to our energy. And if our emotional wellbeing is important to us, we don't want to be left behind in that department either. Here in this chapter you will find a means to give yourself both an energetic boost as well as a renewed state of emotional wellbeing.

Super Energy Boosting Diffuser

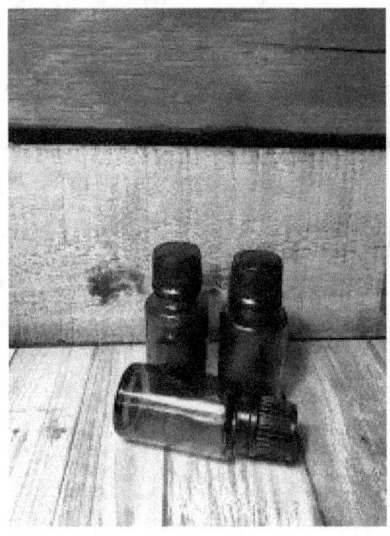

Energy is in desperate demand. We seek it out in our coffee and—even worse—we seek it out in chemically laden energy drinks. And we seek it in large quantities. Through these products we try to bottle up our energy and save it for a rainy day. But don't take another sup of that Red Bull, because we have a super energy boosting diffuser ready and waiting for you!

Here are the exact ingredients:

5 drops of lemon essential oil

5 drops of rosemary essential oil

5 drops of eucalyptus essential oil

5 drops of lime essential oil

3 drops of peppermint essential oil

2 cups of water

This blend brings us the motherload of energy! To get started, get out a large bowl and ad 2 cups of water. Follow this by adding your 5 drops of lemon oil, your 5 drops of rosemary oil, your 5 drops of eucalyptus oil, and your 5 drops of lime oil.

Stir everything together well and allow to sit out at room temperature just long enough for the ingredients to settle in. Once the main ingredients have settled in place, add your 3 drops of peppermint oil on top, give it a good stir and then transfer to your diffuser. You are going to want to allow this potent mix to diffuse through a wide area of your home for at least a few hours. After that you will be good to go.

Mood Boosting Diffuser

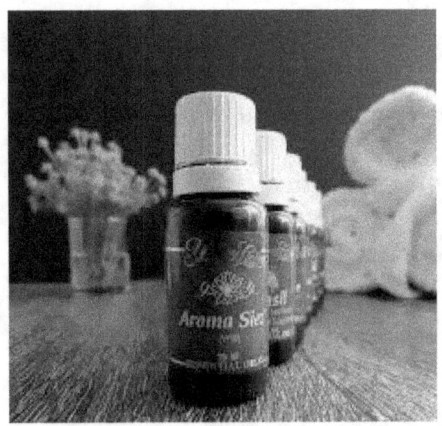

We could all use a little something special to boost our mood from time to time. And this mood boosting diffuser doesn't let you down!

With a powerful blend of eucalyptus oil, lemon oil, rosemary and frankincense, your mood is as good as gold.

Here are the exact ingredients:

2 drops of eucalyptus essential oil

4 drops of frankincense essential oil

2 drops of lemon essential oil

4 drops of rosemary essential oil

This mood booster is just what the aromatherapist ordered! Take out a large mixing bowl and add your cup of water followed by your 2 drops of eucalyptus oil. Stir this together well and drain any excess from the bowl.

After you have done this go ahead and add your 4 drops of frankincense oil, your 2 drops of lemon oil, and your 4 drops of rosemary oil. Proceed to stir everything together, before leaving bowl on the counter to settle for a moment. After settling, pour the mix into your diffuser and enjoy!

Cool Calming Diffuser

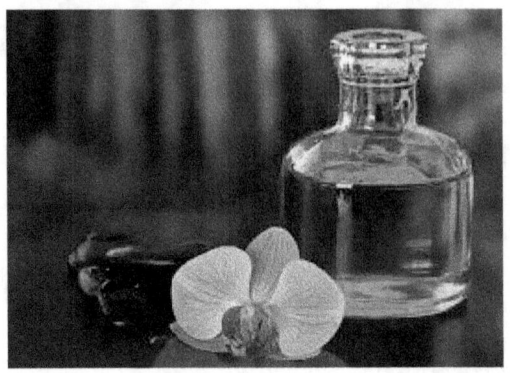

Do you feel like you could use a cool down this summer? Well don't worry my friends because we have the best cool calming diffuser on the block. Check out this fantastic diffuser recipe and you won't be disappointed!

Here are the exact ingredients:

2 drops of rose essential oil

4 drops of lavender essential oil

4 drops of grapefruit essential oil

4 drops of frankincense essential oil

1 cup of water

To get this one started, you will need to take out a large mixing bowl or container and add your 2 cups of water followed by your 4 drops of frankincense. Stir these ingredients together to create a basic base substrate on which the other oils will blend into.

Having that said, once you have created your water/frankincense oil base go ahead and add your 2 drops of rose oil, your 4 drops of lavender oil, and then your 4 drops of grapefruit oil.

Stir these ingredients together and soon you will have a potent citrus and flowery smelling blend, pleasing to the nose just as well as it is pleasing to your general mood.

This mixture could actually be inhaled as is, straight from the bowl, but in order to have the most potent effect you should place the mix into a diffuser and breathe in the aroma slowly, over the next few hours. Pretty soon you will feel invigorated, cool, calm, and completely collected. Here's to a great summer everybody!

Extra Boost Diffuser

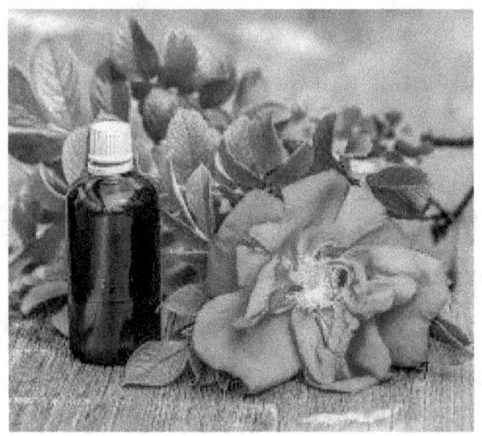

Do you ever feel like you need just a little bit of a boost in order to get going? Well don't worry my friends because this extra boost diffuser gives you just the kick in the pants that you need in order to have a happy and successful day! Go ahead and give this extra boost diffuser a try!

Here are the exact ingredients:

2 drops of clove essential oil

4 drops of clary sage essential oil

4 drops of tangerine essential oil

2 drops of thyme essential oil

2 cups of water

This special mixture will most certainly give you a good boost. Just one whiff and your afterburners will be revved up and ready to take off! So, without further ado, let's get the ball rolling. Start off by depositing your 2 cups of water into a large bowl or plastic, Tupperware container.

Follow this step by adding your 4 drops of clary sage oil, your 4 drops of tangerine oil, and your 2 drops of clove oil. Stir these ingredients together and allow them to settle in place. Next, add your 2 drops of thyme oil to the top, and stir everything together one final time. After you have done this you can deposit the mixture into your diffuser.

Try to place the diffuser into a centralized place in the home so that you can breathe in the aroma all throughout your day. The effects of this diffuser blend will be felt almost immediately. So, what are you waiting for? Go ahead and give yourself the extra boost you need!

Conclusion: You've Just Got to Love Diffusers!

Diffusers are wonderful instruments of well-being. I can still remember the first time that I started to use diffusers. It was actually recommended by my family physician due to the chronic asthma that I was suffering.

My breathing was getting pretty bad and the old traditional methods of treatments were no longer seeming to help. Growing weary of being prescribed inhalers and nebulizers and having to deal with all the potential side effects that came with them; I decided to go the natural route.

And when I did, I was completely amazed. After just a few sessions with a special diffuser blend, my asthma as well as any and all other allergy symptoms disappeared. It was at this point that I began to look into essential oil combinations and diffusers a little more carefully.

After experimenting a bit, I learned that there was a wide variety of recipes that could be concocted and placed inside a diffuser to treat just about any malady known to man.

This is not hype or hyperbole, this is the truth! I was able to not only cure my asthma through aromatherapy but I was also able to calm my nerves, give myself a boost of energy, and lift my mood. I hope that the blends provided here in this book help you to do the same.

Because when it comes to the essential oil blends provided in this guide, there really is a little something here for everyone. I've said it once, and I've said it twice, but saying it one more time won't make it any less nice—you've just got to love the healing power that diffusers can provide! Thank you for reading!